# How To Get What You Need From Your Doctor's Visit…

# The 7 Questions You Need To Know

*By Kevin Cuccaro, D.O.*

<u>Disclaimer:</u> The mission of Straight Shot Health is to provide health information that is interesting, easy to read but, most importantly, useful.

Because the more you know about your own health and the healthcare system the better decisions you can make.

But please remember the information contained within is informational only. It does not imply a medical relationship or replace a medical relationship with your healthcare provider.

# <u>Notes on Terminology Used in "The 7 Questions You Need To Know…"</u>

Since the most common reason people visit their doctor is for pain I will use that term often. However, the "7 Questions" are also useful for things like rashes, bruises or other things that might not be painful. So sometimes I'll use words like "health problem" or "health complaint" instead of "pain."

Also, since physicians perform most healthcare visits I will use the term "doctor" or "physician" rather than "healthcare provider" or "medical provider."

Again, if you don't have a physician as your "healthcare provider," the principles behind the "7 Questions" are the same.

Lastly, 30% of physicians (and growing) are female. Rather than be gender neutral I'll alternate between "he" & "she" throughout.

Thanks for your understanding!

~ Kevin Cuccaro, D.O.

# Table of Contents

# Introduction

## Why You Need to Know 7 Simple Questions Before Your Doctor's Appointment

**Let's get started with a quick question.**

How much time did your doctor spend with you on your last visit?

I'm not talking about how much time you spent checking in at the front desk…

Or waited in the office…

Or spoke with the medical assistant…

But direct face-to-face time with your doctor?

If you were lucky you had about 15 minutes with him.

If you were REALLY lucky you might have had 30 minutes.

More commonly you had less than 10 minutes. [1, 2]

And in that brief amount of time you needed to explain your problem, answer follow-up questions from your physician, be examined, and discuss what to do next.

*In 10 minutes or less.*

Difficult? Yep.  Unsatisfying? Absolutely.

Effective? Well…it depends on 'what' is being treated.

If you're having a heart attack and you're rushing through the emergency department…

we (as in medical professionals) can do a decent job.

But MOST physician visits are not for emergencies.

Instead they are to *Evaluate, Reassure* and *Educate*.

*Evaluate* the health problem and determine whether it may be "serious" or not.[a]

*Reassure* us on the next step to take. This could be testing, medication or just time to allow the body to heal.

*Educate* us on how to improve and feel better through better diet, exercise, or stress reduction.

But to *Evaluate* AND *Reassure* AND *Educate* takes <u>Time</u>.

Time our healthcare system doesn't provide for.

Knowing this we can choose to do a couple of things:

---

[a] We will touch on "serious" in Question #1

> 1) We could moan and groan about how little time doctors spend with patients… all the different reasons for this… how "unfair" it is… how "someone" needs to do something… etc. etc. etc.

**OR**

> 2) We could make sure the time we spend with our doctor—*no matter how much or how little*—is focused intently on the reason for the visit.

Option 1 will require a major overall of the healthcare system. Even if those changes started tomorrow (and they aren't) it would be a long time before any of us noticed improvement.

Waiting for Option 1 will not help us now or anytime soon.

But if we choose Option 2 we can benefit from it now.

This short book is to help you with Option 2.

It gives you seven important questions to think about BEFORE you see your doctor.

Even better you can have these seven questions written down and ready BEFORE your appointment.

This makes the most of the precious time you spend face-to-face with your doctor. It gives you more time for *evaluation, reassurance and education*.

So you can get the answers you <u>need</u> by the end of your visit.

Another important point!  This book is NOT just about answering seven questions.  It's also about how to *think* through these questions. This is important because each question builds upon the previous.

Confused?   Don't worry, I'll provide examples on how to do this throughout the book.

Then answering the questions should be faster and easier for you.

But if something still isn't clear let me know. Up-to-date contact information is available at StraightShotHealth.com.  Your feedback will help future editions of this book be clearer and more useful to those who need it.

Also, feel free to mark up this book and write in it. The margins are wide for a reason. You may find your own questions (or sub-questions) that work for you or help with your specific medical problem.

For example, some conditions are associated with frequent medical visits. Using this book as a 'note book' may help you keep track of previous visits, past treatments, new questions to ask, etc.

Finally, if you'd like a downloadable "7 Question" form you can print and use for future doctor's visits go to: StraightShotHealth.com/7Questions

# Why Should I Bother Listening To You Dr. Cuccaro?

Great question!

When it comes to your health you should ALWAYS question the source.

Why? Because there is a lot of bad information out there.

Especially now.

So I want you to understand who I am and what is important about this simple book.

Then you can decide for yourself whether you should listen to me.

Here's the story…

I'm a Doctor of Osteopathic Medicine (D.O.) and graduate of the Chicago College of Osteopathic Medicine.[b]

---

[b] D.O.'s and M.D.'s are both medical doctors. We all prescribe medicines, do

I trained in Anesthesiology at the University of Chicago and performed a Fellowship (more training) in Pain Medicine at The University of Michigan.

After my training, I served as an anesthesiologist and pain physician in the United States Navy. I also served as Assistant Program Director of the Pain Medicine Fellowship at San Diego's Naval Medical Center.

Finally, I practiced as a pain physician for a civilian medical group.

However, I slowly realized our healthcare system isn't about health at all.

In fact, there is a huge disconnect between what we do in healthcare and what people need. [3, 4, 5, 6, 7]

---

surgery, pass a bunch of tests and have medical licenses.

There are still D.O.'s and M.D.'s who say we are different. But I've trained and practiced with both and I can't tell who is who until I see the initials.

This is especially true in my specialty of 'Pain Medicine' where I often see people putting profits before patients. [8]

However, you can't simply ignore our healthcare system because all of us, at some point, will need *Evaluation* of a health problem.

If not for ourselves then for a loved one.

So how do you get the *evaluation* when needed but stay safe from a system built around 'doing things' to you?

You prepare.

And that all starts with making sure you're ready for your doctor's appointment.

# How Can These Questions Help Me?

Like I said in the introduction these questions are to help you get the most out of your doctor's appointment.

Sometimes when we go to our doctor we know we just feel "bad." We schedule the appointment. We wait. We're hopeful we'll feel better when we're through.

Then we see our doctor. She asks, "Why are you here today?"

And we don't know how to answer.

We know we don't feel well but we can't explain it…especially now since we're under pressure.

Not a good feeling and it is frustrating.

But the solution is easy.

Run through these questions first. You'll find them easier when you're not having a time-strapped doctor breathing down your neck.

Then at your appointment you'll have your answers all ready to go.

You'll be able to give powerful and important information to your doctor.

Information which helps them figure out…

- The organ system that might be involved (your heart, lungs, stomach, etc.).

- The possible cause of your problem.

- What may be worsening your pain.

- And others…

Your doctor WANTS and NEEDS to know your answers to these questions so she can help you.

So you're helping her…to help you…creating a win-win situation.

Going through these questions beforehand also helps you develop answers that are clear and *to the point.*

*Clear* answers provide "just the facts".

*To the point* answers are "short and sweet."

Long answers aren't what you want. In fact, each answer should only take a few words or, at most, a sentence or two.

You want to provide clear and to the point information FIRST.

THEN, later, you can provide more details.

# Start Here First: Your Number One Concern

Before you start on the "7 Questions" you must first know one thing:

## What are you seeing your doctor for?

This is known in medical talk as your "Chief Complaint." It's the <u>main</u> reason you are in your doctor's office.

It should take you less than 5-10 words to say or write. You can, and should, use your own words.

Examples of Chief Complaint's for new health problems are things like:

*"I have back pain", "I've got a cold", "My nose is runny" or*
*"My throat feels like I swallowed sand paper".*

Your Chief Complaint for past health problems would be whatever you're checking up on like:

*"Check up on [blood pressure, diabetes, sore throat, etc.]"*

Your Chief Complaint tells your doctor a few things.

First it tells him why you are in his office.

Next, your Chief Complaint starts him thinking about potential reasons for your problem.

Finally, your Chief Complaint focuses your doctor's attention on what is concerning to you.

What do I mean by focus his attention? Well doctors are kind of like mechanics.

There are some "classic cars" out there that have unique and interesting features.

When the owner brings his "classic car" in to see his mechanic, those unique and interesting features may be very interesting to the mechanic.

But those fascinating features might have *nothing* to do with why the car owner brought his car to the mechanic.

Unless the owner keeps the mechanic focused on what is concerning to HIM about HIS car... he may not get the answers he wants.

It is the same way in healthcare.

Some diseases are very interesting (yes... doctors are weird).

You could have an interesting disease but it might have <u>nothing</u> to do with why you're seeing your doctor today.

But if your doctor doesn't know this he will use all his time talking about the interesting disease.

A written Chief Complaint (and the 7 Questions) keeps your doctor focused on what is most important to YOU—Not them.

# What if You Have Multiple Concerns?

If you have more than one "Chief Complaint" you must know which will be your "#1 Chief Complaint" for <u>this</u> visit.

Like we discussed before, time is limited.

There is a good chance you will only have time to talk about one thing during your appointment.

Fair or not fair, right or wrong, it's the nature of the beast.

So you need to decide in advance what is your main reason you are seeing your doctor. This way your most important problem is addressed.

If you do have more than one health complaint write each one down. Have a "Chief Complaint" and go through the "7 Questions" for each.

But start your visit with your "#1 Chief Complaint."

Get through that one first. Then if there is time you can start on the next.

This is especially important if you are coming in for a new health complaint but you also have old health problems.

If your old health problem is *not the reason you're visiting your doctor right now* don't start there!

Here's an example: You have a new rash on your toes and you have had back pain for ten years.

The rash is new and you are very concerned. Your back pain hasn't changed but it still irritates you.

What would your Chief Complaint be?

In most cases it would be your rash. You've never had it before and you are worried.

So start your appointment with what is most important to you first—*your rash!*

The old back pain can wait until after the rash is looked at.

I've talked to people who've gone to their doctor, had an appointment and left without ever having their "#1 Chief Complaint" discussed.

Why? Because their doctor never knew what their "#1 Chief Complaint" was.[c]

So make sure to focus on what is <u>your</u> main reason you are seeing your doctor.

Then your doctor doesn't need to try and read your mind… and we are awful mind readers.

---

[c] As a doctor I've done this as well. If the patient doesn't make it clear what is most important to them…I have to choose for them. Unless my guess is correct neither of us is satisfied when the visit is through.

# Question #1:

## When did your problem or pain begin?

Did it start yesterday, last week… or last year?

This question helps figure out how **acute** or **chronic** your Chief Complaint is.

It also helps your doctor determine if you have an **emergency** or **urgency**.

Let's talk about emergencies and urgencies first…

An **emergency** requires action now or something horrible could happen (loss of life or limb).

Examples of emergencies are heart attacks, strokes, flesh-eating bacteria, broken bones sticking out of your body, etc.

The stuff you see on the news.

If you have an emergency things are bad and getting worse fast.

This is why we have emergency departments. Emergency departments were designed so you can be seen and treated quickly. [9]

Luckily, true emergencies are rare.

If you're wondering why there are long waits in emergency departments…

…it's because most of the people there are experiencing *urgencies*—not *emergencies*.

An *urgency* is a health problem that may need treatment because it could worsen.

Or it might just be very uncomfortable.

*Urgencies* are *not* likely to kill you or cause you to lose an arm or leg in the next few minutes, hours or days (like emergencies can).

*Urgencies* can be things like coughs, colds, cuts, muscle sprains, rashes etc.

Most urgencies will get better on their own, with or without any care from doctors.

What your doctor is looking for is to see if your urgency is something that may:

- Get worse over time without treatment (ex. Some infections).

- Needs simple care to promote healing (ex. Splints, casts, stiches).

- Just needs to be watched closely to see if it improves on it's own.

Make sense?

Now let's talk about the difference between *acute* and *chronic* health problems.

*Acute* problems usually (but not always) occur quickly. They can develop in minutes, hours or days. They can be very painful or uncomfortable.

"New" health complaints are acute problems.

*Chronic* problems have been around for a while (weeks, months or years). They can be very uncomfortable… or you might not notice them much.

They are "old" health complaints.

Basically the question comes down to…

# Is Your Chief Complaint New or Old???

This difference is important because *most* emergencies or urgencies come from acute health problems.

For example, if you've had your health problem for months or years but it hasn't changed (i.e. chronic)… it is less likely to worsen quickly or cause significant harm in the next few days or weeks.

With chronic health problems you *usually* have time. Time to order tests, try new treatments, or change your diet and exercise.

*Acute* (new) health problems are trickier.

Why?

Because while most health complaints we experience are not life threatening and they often get better over time without any sort of treatment…

…there are some that *COULD* be very harmful.

Figuring out the difference between "could be harmful" and "probably not harmful" is why you see a doctor.

Your doctor is trying to decide:

> A. Does this health problem require treatment to help your body heal?

> B. Is this health problem likely to get better on its own with or without any treatment?

This is so important I'm going to repeat it again…

*Your doctor is trying to determine **if** your pain or problem is something that **requires** treatment with drugs or surgery.*

Why this distinction?

Because many health problems will get *better* over time on their own <u>without</u> any treatment at all.

Also, there are health complaints that we doctors make *worse* <u>with </u>too much medical care. [3, 10, 11, 12, 13]

The key to good healthcare is to determine which is which.

In Summary, Question #1 determines:

***Emergencies*** vs. ***Urgencies***.

And

**Acute** or **Chronic** health problems.

This question helps your doctor decide:

- Does your health problem need "help" to heal (i.e. if pills or surgery will help)?

- Are any tests or x-rays needed?

- Does your health problem need to be watched closely (i.e. schedule a follow-up appointment)?

- Will "Time and Chicken Soup"
  be all you need (i.e. your health
  problem should get better on its
  own... like most colds do)?

# Question #2:

## Do you feel your problem or pain all the time or only occasionally?

Basically, since your pain started, do you always have it (***constant***) or does it come and go (***intermittent***)?

For example, maybe you woke up with stomach pain and it hasn't stopped.

In this case your stomach pain has been there ***constantly*** since it started.

Here's another example: You have had headaches for five years. You don't have them all the time. In fact, you only have them in the late evenings after being on the computer all day long.

In this case your headaches are occurring ***intermittently*** since they began.

Let's use these two examples (stomach pain and headache) and put together a quick response for each using the first two questions and Chief Complaint:

> 1. "I have a stomachache. It began three weeks ago. My stomachache woke me up from sleep and hasn't gone away since."

> 2. "My headaches began five years ago. I don't have them all the time. They usually start in the late evenings and are more common if I've been using the computer all day."

So far so good? Do you see how much information a few short sentences can provide?

Let's look at them again…

*"I have a stomachache. It began one week ago. My stomachache woke me up from sleep and hasn't gone away since."*

What does this tell your doctor?

It tells her what you're seeing her for today: The Chief Complaint is "Stomachache."

Your answer to Question #1 tells her when and how it started: It woke you up from sleep one week ago.

Your answer to Question #2 tells her it is a constant pain because your stomachache hasn't gone away.

What about for the headache example?

*"My headaches began five years ago. I don't have them all the time. They usually start in the late evenings."*

Chief Complaint? Headache.

Question 1: When did your pain begin? Five years ago.

Question 2: Do you have headaches all the time or only occasionally? Intermittently (or occasionally).

Those three sentences said slowly take only seconds to say.[d]

------

[d] 6.5 seconds for the first description and 6

Yet every word provides important information to your doctor.

---

seconds for the headache when I timed myself.

# Question #3:

## Where do you feel your pain or problem on or in your body?

Sometimes the answer to this question isn't as easy as you might think.

To help, try to think of it this way:

<u>Is there a "Point of Maximum Intensity?"</u>

> A "Point of Maximum Intensity" is a spot you can point to with your finger. That spot would be where you feel most of your pain.

> For rashes or other non-painful problems the "Point of Maximum Intensity" would be where most of the rash is located.

<u>If there is not a "Point of Maximum Intensity":</u>

Is there more than one place on your body your health complaint is found (like both your elbows and hands)?

OR

Does your entire body hurt or does your rash cover your whole body?

If your health problem does involve most of your body try to remember if it started from one particular spot. Then make sure tell your doctor where that starting point was.

# Question #4:

## Does your pain or problem move or stay in one place?

This question builds on to question #3.

It is used a lot for pain problems BUT it can be useful for other health complaints too.

First I'll explain how this question can help if you have pain. Then we'll talk about how it can help if you aren't having pain.

What your doctor wants to know is if you experience pain that…

> ***Moves*** from one area to another without leaving any painful sensations behind?

> ***Shoots*** down or up from one place? Like from your neck down into your arm?

Or *Stays* in the same place all the time (i.e. no shooting pains and no sensations that move around)?

Here are some examples for each.

- *Moving:* Belly pains are often *Moving* type pains. You may have a dull ache in one area of your belly but it doesn't stay there. Throughout the day it might move from upper part of your belly to the lower or from the left side to the right side.

  When moving pains move they tend to pick up all their painful bits with them. They don't leave much (if any) painful spots behind.

  This can also be seen with things like bruising or rashes. The rash may start in one area then move to another location on your body (while the place where the rash started from improves).

- *Shooting:* These pains start in one area but then shoot or radiate from there. Sometimes the shooting pain can very painful—

more painful than the area it started from—but not last long.

They're like little "lightning bolts" or "electric shocks."

"Sciatica" is an example of a shooting pain. People often experience it in the back, which then shoots down into a leg.

- **Stays:** Pain that **stays** doesn't shoot or move. The pain may stay in the same spot for most of the time (It's *constant*… from question #2). Sometimes these pains will come and go (*intermittently*) but they are always in the same place.

  Headaches that occur in the same area are good examples. Back pain without "sciatica" often stays in one place and doesn't change.

How your pain acts (shoots, moves or stays in the same place) helps your doctor think about things that may be associated with your pain.

So use this opportunity to describe exactly how your pain acts, like:

*"Most of my pain is here (point to hip) but when I move like this (demonstrate movement) it shoots into my knee..."*

* * *

Let's summarize the first four questions using our examples of stomachache and headache. Here are what the descriptions could be by answering the first four questions:

1. "I have a stomachache. It began one week ago. My stomachache woke me up from sleep and hasn't gone away since. Most of my stomachache is here **[points with one finger]** but sometimes it moves over here **[points with one finger]**.

2. "My headaches began five years ago. I don't have them all the time. They usually start in the late evenings and last until I go to sleep. They feel like a tight band squeezing my entire head and they don't move."

# Question #5:

## How does your pain feel and how uncomfortable is it?

Sounds simple.

Yet this question can be frustrating to answer if you haven't thought about it.

But it is very important. So we're going to spend some time going through it.

Ready?

Basically your doctor wants to know the *Quality* (the feeling) and the *Quantity* (the intensity) of your health complaint.

We'll start with *Quantity*.

*Quantity* is "how much" discomfort or pain you're feeling.

We measure this with a simple scale of numbers or words.

A number scale could be "0-10".

A word scale could use "mild, moderate, medium, strong, and unbearable (like hot sauce)".

Both types of scales work fine. You just need to use the same scale (words or numbers) consistently.

Number scales like "0-10" are used most often. So I'll describe how to best use a "0-10" scale.

For your scale to work you need to know what your boundaries are. Your boundaries are what is your "0 (no pain)" and what is your "10 (unbearable pain)"?

These boundaries help tell your doctor how "intense" or "how much" pain you're experiencing.

Here's an example of a pain scale from 0-10 with easy to understand boundaries:

***"On a scale from 0-10 where '0' is no pain***

Pretty gruesome BUT it provides easy to understand boundaries.

You know what a '0' is. You can imagine what a '10' could be. With these boundaries you can figure out how your pain fits between them.

Your doctor can now "measure" how much pain you are having. It also helps him see if you're improving or not if you have a follow up visit.

**Very Important**: Pain is not the same for everyone. Your pain is unique to you. It cannot be compared to anyone else's pain— Only your own!

I've had patients try to imagine what their pain would be for someone else. I've also seen patients try to scale their pain by what they think other people's pain scales are.

It doesn't work. You can only compare your pain to… your pain.[e]

You also don't need to try and compare your pain because the "number" by itself isn't very important. What is important is *how your number moves up or down your scale with time or with treatment.*

Okay, enough about **Quantity**. Let's talk about pain **Quality**.

**Quality** *(how it feels)* can be harder to describe than **Quantity** *(how much)*.

Why?

Because you need to bring out your descriptive words.

How does it *feel*?

Does it feel like "a million bees buzzing in my ears"?

---

[e] Geek alert: Pain is what is known as a Quale (plural Qualia). A Quale is a personal experience. Qualia are difficult, if not impossible, to measure between people because each of us experiences things differently.

Does it feel like "an elephant is standing on my chest" (the classic description of a heart attack)?

Is it shocking, tingling, burning, aching, dull, sharp, stabbing, squeezing...?

Does it feel like "lightning" or "liquid fire running over your legs?"

Or maybe "...like I have an alien inside my belly which is trying to bust out!"

Be specific and descriptive when answering how your discomfort feels.

Now, and this is important, saying it "hurts" or it's "just painful" provides little useful information.

Your doctor will know you feel something wrong but that's it.

Describing how your pain feels though helps yourself and your doctor in a few ways.

First, descriptive words help your pain "stick" into your doctor's brain. If you have a follow up visit or phone call, your description of your pain can help her remember you easier. [14]

The other benefit of descriptive words is they help your doctor remember her past experiences.

After 7-10+ years of medical education there are lots of 'past experiences' for your doctor to remember. This doesn't even include the number of years your doctor has been practicing medicine. So she may have treated patients in the past with a similar pain or problem.

When you describe your pain or problem clearly and use descriptive words you're helping her remember those experiences that help her to remember what worked then or what didn't.

That's powerful stuff!

* * *

Here's where we are with our examples after five questions:

1.  "I have a stomachache. It began one week ago. My stomachache woke me up from sleep and hasn't gone away since. Most of my stomachache is here **[points with one finger]** but sometimes it moves over here **[points with one finger]**. My pain is a 5 out of 10 right now. The lowest my pain has been is a 3 and the worst it has been was a 7. My belly feels dull and achy."

2.  "My headaches began five years ago. I don't have them all the time. They usually start in the late evenings and last until I go to sleep. *They feel like a tight band squeezing my entire head and they don't move.* When I have the pain in the evenings it is usually around a 4 out of 10. The worst they've ever been is an 8 out of 10."

*Example number two also shows how describing the location of the pain (Question #3) can sometimes combine with the feeling of the pain (Question #5).*

# Question #6:

## What makes your problem or pain feel better & what makes it worse?

There will *almost always* be at least ONE thing that helps you feel better. There will also *almost always* be at least ONE thing that makes you feel worse.

What are they?

Here are some examples for pain if you're stuck…

Do movements increase your pain? Sitting, standing, walking, running, bending, twisting, or something else?

Be as specific as possible.

Instead of just saying "Sitting makes it worse" try to say "When I sit in hard chairs with my legs crossed it hurts."

If you hurt when you're walking describe what you're walking on: Grass, sand, dirt, concrete?

Maybe your pain only happens when you bend forward and touch your toes… or when you bend backward?

Whatever it is be specific.

Be just as specific when describing what helps your pain feel better.

Does your back feel better after you've been walking around for a while? How long? What are you doing as you walk?

Does your stomachache go away after you've drunk milk? Or when you're not eating? What foods help your stomach? What foods make it worse? How soon does the pain start after you eat? Etc. etc. etc.

Did you use some ointment on your rash and it seemed to get better for a couple of days? What kind of ointment? How often?

*[**Important point:** If you have used some medication or ointment bring it with you to your doctor's appointment.]*

Describing what makes your problem or pain feel better and what makes it feel worse is INCREDIBLY important! It hints at what may be associated with your pain as well as potential treatment options.

**Don't miss this opportunity!**

Don't say, "I don't know."

If you haven't tried anything say, "I haven't tried anything."

Don't say, "Nothing helps." It is not likely you've tried *everything* possible.

Instead describe exactly what you tried that DIDN'T work.

This can be hard to remember especially the more specific you are!

But that is why it is useful to think about these questions <u>before</u> you go see your doctor!

They help you figure out exactly how your pain feels to you.

They help you think about the nitty gritty details of your pain you may have forgotten.

They get you to think of things that might be important for your doctor to hear… but could get missed in a rushed appointment.

They help you to take control of your health.

* * *

Here's where we are with our examples after six questions:

1. "I have a stomachache. It began one week ago. My stomachache woke me up from sleep and hasn't gone away since. Most of my stomachache is here **[points with one finger]** but sometimes in moves over here **[points with one finger]**. My pain is a 5 out of 10 right now. The lowest my pain has been is a 3 and the worst it has been was a 7. My belly feels dull and achy. Eating makes my belly hurt worse—solid foods are the worst but even liquids like soup or water hurt. Lying down helps my pain especially if I lie on my side and pull my legs up."

2. "My headaches began five years ago. I don't have them all the time. They usually start in the late evenings and last until I go to sleep. They feel like a tight band squeezing my entire head and they don't move. When I have the pain in the evenings it is usually around a 4 out of 10. The worst they've ever been is an 8 out of 10. They get worse after I've been using a computer for longer than an hour. They are especially bad if I had to use the computer all day at work. During the week I try to lie down and relax—that usually helps."

# Question #7:

## Is there anything else you noticed around the same time your problem started?

This could be obvious.

Maybe with your cough you've felt hot and feverish or your body is aching too.

But it could be not so obvious.

Like maybe you noticed an odd shaped rash on your hands before your pain began…

Or after you're belly was hurting you noticed your poop was black in color…

Or you're belly hurts and you don't feel like eating anything…

Sometimes we may be so miserable with our pain we don't pay attention to anything else.

But those "anything else's" (if they are not normal for you) can provide your doctor vital clues.

Also, have you done anything that isn't in your normal routine recently?

Have you changed what you eat or eaten new foods? Did you start an exercise program or hike 5 miles? Have you had any weird stumbles or falls? Did you travel (especially out of the country)?

Did you have sex with a new partner?

> *(I inserted this question to be a bit "shocking." Sometimes what we may think is "too personal" can be very important when it comes to your health. It is important to share these with your doctor so they have the information they need to help you.*
>
> *Trust me, by the time we've finished our medical training there is very little that we find "shocking" or embarrassing.*
>
> *It's hard, but try not to let feelings of embarrassment get in the way of helping you find a way to feel well).*

Think like a Private Investigator during this question or like you're playing a game of Clue^(TM)

But instead of "Colonel Mustard in the Library with the Candlestick," you piece together:

*"I ate a potato salad at an outdoor picnic on a really hot day. That evening I started having horrible diarrhea…"*

To be honest, most of the time your health concern won't have any weird "anything else's."

In fact, most of them time your problem or pain will be something routine.

Because if "weird things" were common… they wouldn't be "weird."

Right?

BUT sometimes knowing what else *might* be involved with your health concern—rash, bruise, weight loss or gain, fevers, chills, travel, etc.—could provide your physician with a critical piece of information.

The vital "clue" that answers the big question of "what's wrong with me?"

Kind of like the wrap up at the end of a good murder mystery… without all the murder and mayhem…

Obviously remembering "anything else's" can be a bit tricky—especially if you're thinking back a few months.

But this is another reason why you should think about this before you get to your doctor's office.

* * *

This is the end of the 7 Questions. Here's where we are now with our examples:

1. "I have a stomachache. It began one week ago. My stomachache woke me up from sleep and hasn't gone away since. Most of my stomachache is here **[points with one finger]** but sometimes in moves over here **[points with one finger]**. My pain is a 5 out of 10 right now. The lowest my pain has been is a 3 and the worst it has been was a 7. My belly feels dull and achy. Eating makes my

belly hurt worse—solid foods are the worst but even liquids like soup or water hurt. Lying down helps my pain especially if I lie on my side and pull my legs up. I've noticed that I'm not hungry at all and don't feel like eating. I've also thrown up a few times and I've had a slight temperature. "

2. "My headaches began five years ago. I don't have them all the time. They usually start in the late evenings and last until I go to sleep. They feel like a tight band squeezing my entire head and they don't move. When I have the pain in the evenings it is usually around a 4 out of 10. The worst they've ever been is an 8 out of 10. They get worse after I've been using a computer for longer than an hour. They are especially bad if I had to use the computer all day at work. During the week I try to lie down and relax—that usually helps. I didn't think about this before but I don't get my headaches on vacation even if I use the computer. Also, they first started around the same time I changed jobs."

We now have descriptions that tell your doctor tons of information. Every sentence is important and to the point. Each sentence helps tell the story of your pain to your doctor.

They also only take 30 or 40 seconds to say.

While this is end of the 7 Questions—*and they're the most important*—there is one "bonus question" that is sometimes useful. We'll cover it next.

# The "Bonus" Question

## Have you ever had this before?

The "Bonus Question" helps us remember health problems we may have had years ago but may have forgotten.

It can also help us remember what worked before, or what didn't work.

I've asked this question of patients and had them say…

*"You know what Doc? I had this same pain 5 years ago. It was exactly like this and kind of started in the same way. Back then we did [whatever was done] and it got better [or worse] and then we… etc. etc. etc."*

You get the picture.

Your current health concern could be different. BUT if it feels the SAME, started the SAME way and has the SAME characteristics (where it is, how it feels etc.)….

There is a very good chance it may get better with the SAME treatment you had last time.

[**Side Note:** There are some important caveats here especially for persistent, aka 'chronic,' pain, but that's for another book.]

Answering this question can also help keep you from treatments that didn't work in the past.

Trying to do again what didn't work before is overrated, expensive and…it can hurt you.

How?

Because of something called "intervention bias." Intervention bias basically means that our healthcare system is trained to "do things." [7]

And we prefer to "do things" even when not doing things is a better choice.

Or even when we've already "done things" and they didn't help the first time.

We order lots of labs and x-rays... even in cases when the results won't change your treatment.

We poke people with needles and cut things out... even in cases when the procedure didn't work before or is likely to help now.

So always ask yourself, "Have I felt like this before?"

If you have, make sure you remember what you did back then... and how it all turned out!

Then if your doctor wants to repeat whatever was done last time—*especially if it didn't work*—ask them why?

You should be comfortable with their reasons before you agree to follow whatever they recommend.

# Last Suggestions On How To Use The 7 Questions You Need To Know

Try to write out brief answers for the questions—especially if you get nervous easily!

Make a copy of your answers and give them to the medical assistant when you check in.

If you have more than one pain or health problem make sure you know which is your "number one" concern. Focus on that one first.

Be specific. Avoid long stories or guesses about possibilities.

For example, if you know for sure you noticed your pain week:

> DON'T start off with a story that began months or years ago and finally leads up to your pain starting last week.

DO say, "I noticed it last week."
(Question #1)

If you have friends or family who
have had similar pains and problems
for years.

DON'T spend your time talking
about their health problems.

DO say "I've had my pain constantly
for three weeks." (Question #2).

Remember, you might have only 5-10
minutes to talk with your doctor. Stay
focused on what your *most important*
concern is.

If there is time after focusing on your
"number one" concern… then start on the
next.

# References


[1] Gottschalk A, Flocke SA. Time spent in face-to-face patient care and work outside the examination room. Ann Fam Med. 2005;3(6):488-93.

[2] Block L, Habicht R, Wu AW, et al. In the wake of the 2003 and 2011 duty hours regulations, how do internal medicine interns spend their time?. J Gen Intern Med. 2013;28(8):1042-7.

[3] Hudson B, Zarifeh A, Young L, Wells JE. Patients' expectations of screening and preventive treatments. Ann Fam Med. 2012;10(6):495-502.

[4] Fenton JJ, Jerant AF, Bertakis KD, Franks P. The cost of satisfaction: a national study of patient satisfaction, health care utilization, expenditures, and mortality. Arch Intern Med. 2012;172(5):405-11.

[5] Sirovich BE. How to feed and grow your health care system: comment on "The cost of satisfaction". Arch Intern Med. 2012;172(5):411-3.

[6] Esserman LJ, Thompson IM, Reid B. Overdiagnosis and overtreatment in cancer: an opportunity for improvement. JAMA. 2013;310(8):797-8.


[7] Foy AJ, Filippone EJ. The case for intervention bias in the practice of medicine. Yale J Biol Med. 2013;86(2):271-80.


[8] Roth RS, Geisser ME, Williams DA. Interventional pain medicine: retreat from the biopsychosocial model of pain. Transl Behav Med. 2012;2(1):106-16.


[9] Suter RE. Emergency medicine in the United States: a systemic review. World J Emerg Med. 2012;3(1):5-10


[10] Deyo RA, Mirza SK, Turner JA, Martin BI. Overtreating chronic back pain: time to back off?. J Am Board Fam Med. 2009;22(1):62-8.


[11] Hoffman RM, Couper MP, Zikmund-fisher BJ, et al. Prostate cancer screening decisions: results from the National Survey of Medical Decisions (DECISIONS study). Arch Intern Med. 2009;169(17):1611-8.


[12] Chou R, Deyo RA, Jarvik JG. Appropriate use of lumbar imaging for

evaluation of low back pain. Radiol Clin North Am. 2012;50(4):569-85.

[13] Flynn TW, Smith B, Chou R. Appropriate use of diagnostic imaging in low back pain: a reminder that unnecessary imaging may do as much harm as good. J Orthop Sports Phys Ther. 2011;41(11):838-46.

[14] Heath C, Heath D. Made to Stick, Why Some Ideas Take Hold and Others Come Unstuck. New York: Random House; 2007.

# More Information

If you'd like a copy of 'The 7 Questions'
that you can print out, fill-in-the-blanks, and
take to your next office visit go to:

StraightShotHealth.Com/7questions

It's free and at StraightShotHealth.com
you'll also find podcasts and videos on
various health-related topics (with a special
focus on pain).

Also, if you have questions, feedback, or
stories of how you used 'The 7 Questions'
please feel free to email me at:
DrKevin@StraightShotHealth.Com

Thanks and stay well!

~Kevin Cuccaro, D.O.

# The 7 Questions

First, your chief complaint (Why you are seeing your doctor.):

1. When did your problem or pain begin?

2. Do you feel your problem or pain all the time or only occasionally?

3. Where is your pain or problem on or in your body?

4. Does your pain or problem move or stay in one place?

5. How does it feel and how uncomfortable is it?

6. What makes your problem or pain feel better & what makes it worse?

7. Is there anything else you noticed around the same time?

Bonus Question:  Have you ever had this before?

# About The Author

Dr. Kevin Cuccaro's mission is to transform society's understanding of pain to provide hope and improve patient outcomes.

He frequently speaks on pain and other health-related topics, consults health systems on chronic pain, and has created pain education programs for diverse audiences.

In 2016, the Oregon Health Authority's Transformation Center selected Dr. Cuccaro as a Clinical Innovations Fellow for his innovative work involving pain education in Patient-Centered Primary Care Homes. In 2017, Dr. Cuccaro was appointed to the Oregon Pain Management Commission and serves on the Health Evidence Review Committee's Chronic Pain Task Force.

In addition to systems transformation work, Dr. Cuccaro maintains a small practice in Philomath, Oregon.

To learn more visit: KevinCuccaro.Com